LIFESTYLE RED ALERT

Change Now or Die Early!"

A Wake-Up Call for Those Struggling to Change Their Diet and Exercise Routine

By

Wayne C. Robinson

Disclaimer

The information provided in this book is for educational and informational purposes only and is not intended as medical advice. I am not a medical professional, doctor, or healthcare provider. The content in this book is based on research, personal experience, and general health principles, but it should not be used as a substitute for professional medical diagnosis, treatment, or advice.

If you have any medical concerns, consult a licensed healthcare professional before making any changes to your diet, exercise routine, or lifestyle. If you experience a medical emergency, call 911 immediately or seek urgent medical care.

By reading this book and applying its principles, you assume full responsibility for your own health and actions. The author and publisher are not responsible or liable for any injuries, health complications, or outcomes resulting from the use of the information in this book. Every individual's health situation is unique, and results may vary.

Use this information at your own risk.

Copyright Page
Title: *Lifestyle Red Alert*
Author: *Wayne C. Robinson*

Introduction: The Emergency You're Ignoring

The Harsh Truth: You Are Running Out of Time

Right now, as you read these words, your body is making a decision. It's either healing itself or slowly shutting down. There is no in-between. Every bite of food, every step you do or don't take, every hour you spend sitting instead of moving—these choices are either keeping you alive or pushing you closer to an early grave.

This isn't an exaggeration. This is reality. **Diabetes, heart disease, obesity—these are not just statistics. These are silent killers.** They don't show up suddenly. They creep in, day by day, decision by decision, until one day... it's too late.

- One minute, you feel "fine."
- The next, you're clutching your chest as your heart gives out.
- Or you wake up and can't feel your toes because **diabetes is destroying your nerves.**
- Or you realize your kidneys are failing, your eyesight is dimming, or your legs need to be amputated—all because you **ignored the warning signs.**

Diabetes, Heart Disease, and Obesity: The Silent Killers

More than **700,000 people die from heart disease** every single year in the U.S. alone. That's nearly **one person every 44 seconds.** Diabetes isn't far behind, leading to **kidney failure, blindness, strokes, and amputations** in millions of Americans. These conditions don't just ruin your health—they **steal your time, your energy, your freedom.**

Yet most people **wait until it's too late** to do anything about it. They don't change their diet. They don't exercise. They keep saying:

◈ "I'll start next Monday."

◈ "I just don't have the time."

◈ "I know I should, but I just can't stick with it."

And then one day, **their body makes the choice for them.**

Why Most People Fail to Change (And How to Break the Cycle)

It's not because they don't care. It's because:

1. **They believe they have more time than they do.** (They don't.)
2. **They rely on motivation instead of discipline.** (Motivation fades. Discipline lasts.)
3. **They think small changes won't make a difference.** (They will.)
4. **They're waiting for a doctor's warning instead of acting now.** (By then, it's often too late.)

So how do you **break this cycle**? How do you finally push yourself to **change before you end up in the hospital—or worse, the morgue?**

That's what this book is about.

This Book is Your Final Warning Before It's Too Late

I won't sugarcoat anything. **This is your last wake-up call.**

I'm going to show you:

✔ **How to force yourself to change—no excuses.**

✔ **How to start eating right and exercising—even if you hate it.**

✔ **How to reprogram your mind and habits so you never go back.**

You don't need more information. **You need a plan. You need a push. You need to act NOW.**

This is **your emergency moment.**

Your life is at stake.

If you don't change, you will suffer the consequences.

Turn the page and let's get to work—before it's too late.

Chapter 1: The Truth About Your Body's Deadline

The Science of Deterioration: How Years of Poor Habits Destroy Your Body

Your body is a machine—complex, resilient, and built to sustain life for decades. But just like any machine, **if you neglect it, it will break down.**

Every choice you make—what you eat, how much you move, how you handle stress—either helps your body regenerate **or speeds up its deterioration.**

For years, you may have been:

- Eating **processed, sugar-laden foods** that spike blood sugar and cause inflammation.
- Sitting for **hours on end**, causing poor circulation and muscle loss.
- Consuming **excess alcohol**, overloading your liver and kidneys.
- Ignoring stress, allowing **cortisol to wreak havoc** on your heart, brain, and metabolism.

At first, your body fights back. It **tries to repair itself**, balancing the damage as best it can. But over time, if you keep pushing it past its limits, your body **starts to lose the battle.**

And the scariest part?

Most of the damage happens **silently, without you even realizing it.**

The Silent Killers: High Blood Pressure, Diabetes, Clogged Arteries, Fatty Liver

By the time you **feel** something is wrong, the damage is already extensive. The real threats to your life don't always come with obvious warning signs. They work quietly—until one day, **they strike.**

◈ **High Blood Pressure (The Hidden Time Bomb)**

- It's called the **silent killer** because most people don't even know they have it.
- Causes **heart attacks, strokes, kidney failure, and aneurysms.**
- Often goes unnoticed **until a medical emergency occurs.**

◈ **Type 2 Diabetes (The Sugar Trap)**

- Your blood sugar levels stay too high for too long, leading to **nerve damage, vision loss, and organ failure.**
- Left untreated, diabetes can **cause amputations** and put you at risk for life-threatening infections.
- Nearly **40 million** people in the U.S. have diabetes—most could have prevented it with lifestyle changes.

◈ **Clogged Arteries (Your Body's Slow-Motion Heart Attack)**

- Years of **unhealthy eating and lack of exercise** cause fatty deposits to build up in your blood vessels.
- Eventually, a **blockage forms—leading to a heart attack or stroke.**
- The worst part? **Most people don't know their arteries are clogged until they collapse.**

◈ **Fatty Liver Disease (The Ticking Clock on Your Organs)**

- Your liver is responsible for **detoxifying your body**—but when it's overloaded with processed foods and alcohol, **fat starts to build up in**

it.

- A fatty liver leads to **cirrhosis, liver failure, and even liver cancer.**
- **No symptoms appear early on—until it's too late.**

The Myth of Feeling Fine: Why Your Body Can Be Dying Even If You Don't Feel Sick

You might be thinking:

⟐ "I feel fine, so I must be healthy."

⟐ "I don't have any pain, so nothing is wrong."

⟐ "I can still do my daily activities, so I must be okay."

This is the **biggest lie** your body tells you.

Most chronic diseases **don't cause symptoms right away.** That's why people **collapse from heart attacks** without warning. That's why diabetes **destroys nerves and organs before people even realize they have it.**

By the time you "feel" something is wrong, **it's often too late.**

Doctors don't see the healthiest patients in hospitals. They see the ones who thought they were fine—until their **bodies betrayed them.**

The Real Statistics: How Many People Die Unnecessarily Every Single Day

Let's look at the hard numbers:

- **Heart disease kills 700,000 Americans every year.** That's **one death every 44 seconds.**
- **Diabetes is responsible for nearly 100,000 deaths annually.**
- **Obesity-related diseases kill over 300,000 people every year.**
- **Stroke is the 5th leading cause of death in the U.S.**

The tragic truth? **Most of these deaths were preventable.**

People aren't dying from accidents. **They're dying from years of bad habits.** They're dying **because they didn't change when they had the chance.**

Your Body's Deadline Is Closer Than You Think

This is not a warning for "someday." This is a **crisis happening right now.**

- **If you're overweight, your heart is already under stress.**
- **If you eat poorly, your arteries are already clogging.**
- **If you never exercise, your body is already breaking down.**

Every single day you continue on the same path, **you are accelerating your own deadline.**

But here's the good news: **You have a choice.**

- You can **reverse** many of these conditions.
- You can **prevent** the worst from happening.
- You can **rebuild your health before it's too late.**

This book isn't about waiting for a diagnosis.
It's about **beating the disease before it beats you.**
Your time is running out. What will you do about it?

Chapter 2: Pills Won't Save You

The Illusion of Medication: Why Drugs Don't Cure, They Only Manage

If you're taking pills for **high blood pressure, diabetes, high cholesterol, or any other chronic disease**, let's get one thing straight:

◈ Your medication is not curing you.

Your doctor may have told you that you just need to take a pill every day and you'll be "fine." But the truth is, those pills are **only managing your symptoms—not addressing the root cause.**

Think about it:

- If blood pressure medication **cured** hypertension, why do you have to take it for life?
- If diabetes medication **fixed** your blood sugar issues, why do diabetics keep needing higher doses?
- If cholesterol-lowering drugs **eliminated** the problem, why do so many people on statins still suffer from heart attacks?

The reality is **medication doesn't fix the problem—it just masks it.** It's like putting tape over a broken pipe and hoping it won't leak again.

But here's the part that Big Pharma **doesn't want you to realize**:

Many of these conditions are **reversible**—without pills.

Your blood pressure, blood sugar, cholesterol, and heart health are **all directly impacted by your lifestyle.** Yet instead of teaching you how to fix the root cause, the healthcare system **keeps you dependent on medication.**

Why?

Because **there's too much money to be made in keeping you sick.**

How Big Pharma Profits from Your Lifestyle Diseases

Big Pharma is a **multi-trillion-dollar industry.** And guess what? **Their profits depend on people staying sick.**

Think about it:

◈ If you get **healthy**, you stop needing their drugs.

◈ If you stop needing their drugs, **they lose money.**

◈ So instead of focusing on **prevention**, they sell you **lifelong prescriptions.**

Here's how they keep the cycle going:

They Create Lifelong Customers, Not Cures

- Blood pressure pills, diabetes drugs, cholesterol meds—**these are designed to be taken for life.**
- They don't fix the underlying issue; they just make it **more manageable.**
- Meanwhile, your health continues to decline... meaning **you'll need even more medication over time.**

They Treat Symptoms, Not the Cause

- High blood pressure? Take a pill.
- High cholesterol? Take another pill.
- High blood sugar? Here's some insulin.

Instead of showing you how to fix the real problem—your diet, your lifestyle, your stress—they give you a quick-fix pill.

Why? Because **teaching you how to heal naturally doesn't make them money.**

They Push Doctors to Prescribe Instead of Educate

- Many doctors are trained to **prescribe first, explain later.**
- They're overloaded with patients and **don't have the time** to coach people on lifestyle changes.
- And let's not forget: **Pharmaceutical companies fund medical schools, sponsor research, and pay doctors to promote their drugs.**

The result? **Millions of people stuck on medication for life—when they could have reversed their condition through proper diet, exercise, and lifestyle changes.**

The Real Solution: Prevention, Not Prescription

Here's the hard truth:

◈ **No pill will fix what your lifestyle is destroying.**

If you want real health, you need to **take control of your body.**

You don't have a blood pressure **medication deficiency.**

You don't have a **cholesterol-lowering drug deficiency.**

You don't have a **diabetes pill deficiency.**

You have a lifestyle problem.

And **you** are the only one who can fix it.

So what's the alternative?

Change Your Diet—Now

- Cut out **processed junk, sugar, refined carbs, and trans fats.**
- Eat **real, whole foods—fruits, vegetables, lean proteins, and healthy fats.**
- Lower **your salt and sugar intake** and focus on **nutrient-dense meals.**

Move Your Body—Every Single Day

- You don't need to kill yourself in the gym—**just move.**
- Walk, stretch, lift some weights—**whatever it takes to get your body active.**
- **Sitting all day is a death sentence.**

Take Responsibility for Your Own Health

- Stop waiting for a doctor to save you. **They can't.**
- Stop thinking a pill is the answer. **It's not.**
- Stop making excuses. **Your life is in your hands.**

If you **fix your habits**, your body will heal itself. But if you **keep relying on pills**, you'll stay trapped in the cycle—until one day, your body gives out.

Choose wisely.

Chapter 3: The Painful Reality of What's Coming If You Don't Change

Most people don't change until they have no choice.

They wait until a **doctor looks them in the eye and says, "You need surgery."**

They wait until they **wake up in a hospital bed, wondering what went wrong.**

They wait until their **legs are gone, their vision is fading, or their body has broken down.**

By then, it's too late.

If you don't take action now, your body **will force you to face the consequences**—and when that day comes, there will be no turning back.

Let me introduce you to some people who thought they had "more time" to change... until time ran out.

Real Stories: People Who Ignored Warnings and Paid the Price

◈ "I Never Thought It Would Happen to Me"—Until It Did

James was 52 years old. He was told by his doctor for years to lose weight and exercise. He always said the same thing: **"I'll start next month."**

Then one day, while walking up a flight of stairs, **his heart stopped.**

A major heart attack—right there, in the middle of his office.

They revived him, but the damage was done.

Now he **lives with permanent heart failure.** He takes multiple medications daily, can't walk long distances, and will never get his full health back.

His regret? **He waited too long.**

"I Thought Diabetes Was Just About Sugar"—Then I Went Blind

Lisa, a 45-year-old woman with type 2 diabetes, was prescribed **Metformin and insulin.** She told herself that since she was on medication, she could keep eating what she wanted.

She ignored her doctor's warnings to change her diet.

One morning, **she woke up and couldn't see out of one eye.** A few months later, she lost vision in the other.

Diabetic retinopathy stole her sight. And she could have prevented it—if only she had made changes earlier.

"I Thought I Just Had a Little Numbness"—Until I Lost My Leg

Chris was diagnosed with **diabetes** at 40. He started feeling a tingling in his foot but ignored it. "It's nothing serious," he thought.

But over time, **his foot turned black.**

His doctor told him the blood flow had been cut off due to **diabetic neuropathy.**

The result? **His leg had to be amputated below the knee.**

What's worse? **It didn't have to happen.** If he had changed his diet, exercised, and controlled his sugar intake, he **could have saved his leg.**

Amputations, Blindness, Strokes, and Heart Attacks—What's Next If You Keep Ignoring the Signs

If you're still ignoring your health, **here's what's coming for you:**

◈ **Heart Attack** – Your arteries clog, and suddenly, your heart **stops beating.** If you're lucky, you survive. If not, **your family buries you.**

◈ **Stroke** – Your brain is starved of oxygen, leaving you **paralyzed, unable to talk, and dependent on others.**

◈ **Blindness** – Diabetes destroys your eyes from the inside out. **One day, you wake up and can't see.**

◈ **Amputation** – Poor circulation kills your feet and legs. **Doctors start cutting off parts of your body—first toes, then feet, then legs.**

◈ **Early Death** – One day, your **body just shuts down.** No more second chances. No more time to "start next Monday."

Is this the future you want?

The Financial Cost of Staying Sick: Hospital Bills, Lost Income, Burdening Your Family

Still think your health doesn't matter? Let's talk money.

- The average heart attack patient **spends over $100,000** on medical bills.
- A single stroke **can cost $250,000** in hospital stays, rehab, and long-term care.
- The lifetime cost of diabetes care **exceeds $500,000.**

And if you think **insurance will cover everything, think again.**

◈ **Medications** – You could spend thousands a year on insulin, statins, and blood pressure pills.

◈ **Hospital stays** – The co-pays and deductibles **add up fast.**

◈ **Lost income** – If you're sick, you can't work. If you can't work, **how will you pay your bills?**

◈ **Burden on your family** – Someone will have to **take care of you.** Do you really want your spouse or kids **changing your diapers** because you had a stroke?

Being sick **is expensive.** And most of these costs **are preventable.**

The Emotional Cost: Depression, Low Energy, Poor Quality of Life

Money isn't the only thing you'll lose.

◈ Imagine **waking up every day feeling exhausted, sick, and broken.**

◈ Imagine **not being able to play with your kids or grandkids** because you can't even stand for long.

◈ Imagine **being a burden** to your family—needing help to eat, shower, or even use the bathroom.

That's the reality for **millions of people** who refused to take action until it was too late.

Your body is your home. **If you don't take care of it, you'll lose everything.**

Your Future Is Up to You

◇ You have two choices right now. ◇

Keep ignoring your health. Keep eating the same junk, staying inactive, and waiting for disaster to strike. When it does, you'll remember this chapter—but by then, it will be too late.

Take action NOW. Start changing your habits before your body forces you to.

Which will you choose?

Because the painful truth is this:

Your body doesn't care about your excuses.

It doesn't care if you're "too busy."

It doesn't care if you "don't like healthy food."

It doesn't care if you "hate exercising."

It will break down if you don't take care of it.

The question is: **Will you wait until it's too late—or will you fight for your life now?**

Chapter 4: Why Most People Fail to Change Their Lifestyle

The Psychology of Resistance: Why Your Brain Fights Against New Habits

Change is hard—**not because you lack willpower, but because your brain is wired to resist it.**

Your brain's job is to keep you **safe and comfortable.** It prefers routine because routine means **less effort, less risk, and less uncertainty.**

When you try to make a change—whether it's eating healthier, exercising, or breaking bad habits—**your brain fights back.**

◈ **"This is too hard."**

◈ **"I'll just do it later."**

◈ **"One more cheat meal won't hurt."**

◈ **"I don't feel like it today."**

These thoughts aren't real barriers—they're **mental roadblocks designed to keep you in your comfort zone.**

Why Do Most People Stay Stuck?

◈ **Instant gratification beats long-term rewards** – Junk food gives you instant pleasure, while eating healthy takes longer to show benefits.

◈ **Habits are deeply ingrained** – Your brain prefers repeating the same behaviors rather than learning new ones.

◈ **Fear of failure** – Many people don't start because they're afraid they won't succeed.

◈ **Overwhelm** – Trying to change everything at once feels impossible, so most people don't even try.

But here's the truth: **Your comfort zone is killing you.**

If you don't learn how to **override** your brain's resistance, you'll keep repeating the same patterns **until your body forces you to stop.**

How Society Has Made Junk Food, Laziness, and Quick Fixes the Norm

Look around you. **The world is designed to keep you unhealthy.**

◈ **Fast food commercials** run non-stop, making unhealthy choices seem normal.

◈ **Every store is filled with processed, sugary, and cheap foods.**

◈ **Technology has made life so convenient that people barely move anymore.**

Society encourages:

◈ **Fast food over home-cooked meals.**

◈ **Sitting for hours over physical activity.**

◈ **Medication over lifestyle change.**

◈ **Quick fixes over real solutions.**

The result? **Most people eat poorly, move less, and rely on medication to manage diseases that shouldn't exist in the first place.**

If you want to **break free**, you have to stop following the crowd.

Because here's the reality:

◈ **Most people are sick. Most people are overweight. Most people feel like crap every day.**

Do you really want to be like most people?

If not, you have to reject **the culture of laziness and excuses** and start thinking for yourself.

The "I'll Start Tomorrow" Trap (And How to Break Out of It)

How many times have you said, **"I'll start Monday"** or **"Next month, I'll really commit"?**

This is **one of the biggest lies we tell ourselves.**

Why? Because "tomorrow" never comes.

The cycle looks like this:

You feel guilty about your bad habits.

You promise yourself you'll change—**but not today.**

You keep eating junk, skipping workouts, and avoiding action.

Days turn into weeks, weeks into months... and before you know it, **years have passed.**

This is called **procrastination by false hope.**

You think you're doing something by "planning" to start. But in reality, **you're doing nothing.**

How to Escape the Trap

◈ **Take action immediately.** Not next week. Not next month. **TODAY.**

◈ **Start small.** Don't try to change everything overnight—just focus on **one habit at a time.**

◈ **Remove decision fatigue.** Have a clear plan so you don't waste time "thinking about" what to do.

◈ **Track your progress.** Seeing results keeps you motivated.

If you don't start **now,** you probably never will.

The Power of Identity Change—Stop Calling Yourself "Lazy" or "Stuck"

One of the biggest reasons people fail? **They define themselves by their past habits.**

◈ **"I'm just not the kind of person who eats healthy."**

◈ **"I've always been lazy."**

◈ **"I've never been able to stick with anything."**

If you keep saying these things, **they become your reality.**

Your Identity Shapes Your Actions

◈ If you believe you're lazy, you'll act lazy.

◈ If you believe you have no self-control, you'll make excuses.

◈ If you believe you "can't change," you won't even try.

To truly transform your life, **you need to change how you see yourself.**

Instead of saying **"I'm not disciplined,"** say **"I am building discipline."**

Instead of saying **"I hate exercise,"** say **"I am becoming someone who moves daily."**

Instead of saying **"I'll never be fit,"** say **"I am learning how to take care of my body."**

When you change your identity, **your actions will follow.**

Final Wake-Up Call: No One is Coming to Save You

If you're waiting for the **perfect moment to start, it will never come.**

If you're waiting for **motivation, it will never last.**

If you're waiting for **someone to push you, you're giving away your power.**

⟐ **You are the only one who can change your life.** ⟐

Your brain will resist.

Society will tempt you.

Your old habits will fight back.

But if you don't take control, you already know where you're headed—**straight toward disease, regret, and an early death.**

The choice is simple:

⟐ **Do you want to stay stuck, or do you want to fight for your future?**

If you're ready to break free, **turn the page. It's time to take action.**

Chapter 5: Emergency Action Plan – The 90-Day Lifesaving Formula

◈ This is your emergency intervention. ◈

You don't have time to "ease into it." You don't have months to "figure it out."

If you're reading this, **your body is already running out of time.**

The good news? **You can reverse course—starting today.**

This **90-day plan** is not a diet. It's not a quick fix. **It's your survival guide.**

If you follow it, you'll **lose weight, lower your blood pressure, stabilize your blood sugar, and rebuild your body from the inside out.**

You don't need fancy programs. You don't need expensive supplements. **You just need to commit.**

Step 1: Change Your Diet Today – Not Tomorrow

🔶 **Food is medicine.** What you eat determines whether your body heals—or breaks down.

You don't have to be perfect. **You just have to start.**

The "One Swap at a Time" Method for Instant Progress

Trying to overhaul your entire diet overnight is **a recipe for failure.** Instead, **swap out one bad habit at a time.**

🔶 **Instead of soda → drink water or unsweetened tea.**

🔶 **Instead of white bread → choose whole grain.**

🔶 **Instead of chips → eat nuts or fruit.**

🔶 **Instead of fast food → make a simple home-cooked meal.**

Each swap **moves you closer to health.** And when you commit to it, **it becomes your new normal.**

What to Eliminate Immediately 🔶

Certain foods are **killing you faster than you realize.** The moment you cut them out, **your body starts healing.**

🔶 **Processed sugar** – Spikes blood sugar, fuels diabetes, and increases inflammation.

🔶 **Trans fats** – Found in margarine, fried foods, and processed snacks—**destroys your heart.**

🔶 **Fast food** – Loaded with salt, bad fats, and hidden sugars—**a heart attack on a plate.**

🔶 **Sodas and energy drinks** – Liquid sugar **disguised as "refreshment."**

The Best Foods for Reversing Damage 🔶

🔶 **Dark leafy greens** – Cleans your arteries, lowers blood pressure, and fights inflammation.

🔶 **Healthy fats** – Avocados, nuts, and olive oil **protect your heart and brain.**

🔶 **Clean proteins** – Wild-caught fish, organic chicken, and grass-fed beef **help rebuild muscle and balance blood sugar.**

🔶 **Fiber-rich foods** – Beans, lentils, and whole grains **help prevent diabetes and support digestion.**

◈ **Rule of thumb:** If it came from nature, **eat it.** If it was made in a lab, **leave it alone.**

Step 2: Move Your Body – Even If You Hate Exercise

◈ **Your body was designed to move.** Staying inactive **is killing you.**

The problem? **Most people overcomplicate exercise.** They think they need expensive gym memberships, intense routines, or hours of training.

You don't. **You just need to move—every single day.**

The Simple 15-Minute-a-Day Rule for Beginners

If you're starting from zero, **set a timer for 15 minutes.**

Do **anything active**—walk, stretch, do push-ups, or dance. **Just move.**

You can always **increase later**, but the key is **consistency, not intensity.**

◈ **15 minutes a day = 105 minutes per week = Over 91 hours per year.** That's more than enough to start transforming your health.

Why Walking Can Be More Powerful Than Running

◈♂ Walking **lowers blood pressure, improves circulation, and strengthens your heart.**

◈ It's **gentle on your joints**—perfect if you're overweight or have knee problems.

◈ It **reduces stress and boosts mental clarity.**

◈ Just **30 minutes a day** can **slash your risk of heart disease by 50%.**

How to Exercise Without the Gym

Not a fan of gyms? No problem. Here's how to **build strength and stamina anywhere:**

◈ **Bodyweight exercises** – Squats, push-ups, and lunges require **zero equipment.**

◈ **Movement during screen time** – Do jumping jacks, stretch, or march in place while watching TV.

◈ **Household workouts** – Gardening, cleaning, and carrying groceries **count as exercise!**

◈ **Bike instead of drive** – Every little movement adds up.

◈ **Your goal:** Move every day. **No excuses.**

Step 3: Reset Your Mind for Success

Your body will only change **if your mind changes first.**

Most people fail because **they rely on motivation.** But motivation **comes and goes. Discipline is what keeps you going.**

Why Self-Discipline Is a Muscle (And How to Train It)

Discipline **is not something you're born with.** It's something you **build.**

- The more you **push through discomfort**, the stronger your discipline gets.
- The more you **follow through on commitments**, the more confident you become.
- The more you **stick to small daily actions**, the easier they become.

◈ **Think of it like lifting weights.** At first, it's hard. But the more you do it, **the stronger you get.**

The "Do It Anyway" Method: How to Take Action Even When You Don't Feel Like It

◈ **Don't want to go for a walk? Go anyway.**

◈ **Craving junk food? Eat something healthy instead.**

◈ **Feel like skipping today? Show up for 5 minutes, then decide.**

◈ **Your feelings don't have to control your actions.**

Action leads to motivation, not the other way around.

◈ **The more you take action, the more you'll WANT to keep going.**

Visualizing Your Future Self: Do You Want to Live... or Just Survive?

Take a moment and **imagine your life in 5 years.**

Option 1 **You take control now.**

◈ You feel strong, energetic, and in control of your body.

◈ You avoid expensive medications and hospital visits.

◈ You enjoy time with your family—without worrying about your health.

Option 2 **You do nothing.**

◈ You're overweight, struggling to breathe, and exhausted every day.

◈ You're on multiple medications with painful side effects.

◈ You're facing **serious health complications—or worse.**

Which future do you want?

◈ **Your choices today determine your life tomorrow.**

Final Challenge: Start Today, Not Tomorrow

◈ **You don't need more time. You don't need more information.**

◈ You **just need to start.**

This isn't about willpower. **This is about survival.**

◈ **Your excuses won't save you.**

◈ **Your doctor won't save you.**

◈ **Your family can't save you.**

Only **YOU can save yourself.**

90 days. That's all it takes to turn your life around.

◈ **Start with one food swap today.**

◈ **Move for 15 minutes today.**

◈ **Make one disciplined choice today.**

◈ **Every step you take moves you closer to life... or closer to death.**

Which direction will you choose?

Chapter 6: No More Excuses – Here's How You Stay on Track

LIFESTYLE RED ALERT

By now, you know **what's at stake.** You know how dangerous it is to ignore your health. You know that pills won't save you, and that lifestyle change is your only way out.

But **knowing isn't enough.**

Most people fail **not because they don't understand the risks**, but because **they don't stick with the changes long enough to see results.**

This chapter is about one thing: **staying on track—no matter what.**

Because your success doesn't come from a perfect plan. It comes from **consistency.**

The "Habit Stacking" Method: Making Small Changes That Stick

◈ **The #1 reason most people fail? They try to change too much at once.**

They go from eating junk food every day to **an extreme diet.**

They go from never exercising to **two-hour workouts.**

They go from making no changes to **overhauling their entire lifestyle overnight.**

And after a few days? **They give up.**

Why? **Because it's too much, too fast.**

The solution? Habit stacking.

What is Habit Stacking?

Habit stacking is the process of **attaching new habits to existing ones** so they feel natural.

Instead of **forcing** yourself to create new behaviors from scratch, you **build them into your current routine.**

◈ **Example: Want to drink more water?**

➡ Every time you **brush your teeth, drink a full glass of water.**

◈ **Example: Want to exercise more?**

➡ Every time you **watch TV, do squats or march in place during commercials.**

◈ **Example: Want to eat healthier?**

➡ Every time you **make coffee, grab a healthy snack instead of something processed.**

Start Small, Then Build Up

You don't need **a massive transformation overnight.** You just need **small wins every day.**

◈ **Day 1:** Drink one extra glass of water.

◈ **Day 3:** Walk for 10 minutes.

◈ **Day 7:** Swap fast food for home-cooked meals.

◈ **Day 14:** Add 5 minutes of stretching every morning.

Each change **compounds over time**, until **healthy habits become second nature.**

How to Surround Yourself with the Right Influences

◈ **Your environment determines your success.**

If you surround yourself with **junk food, unhealthy people, and negativity, you'll fail.**

If you surround yourself with **healthy food, supportive people, and motivation, you'll succeed.**

1 Clean Up Your Physical Environment

Make bad habits harder and good habits easier.

◈ **Throw away junk food.** If it's not in your house, you won't eat it.

◈ **Put workout clothes where you see them.** Lay them out the night before.

◈ **Keep water nearby.** Make drinking water as easy as possible.

◈ **Prep healthy snacks in advance.** Convenience beats willpower every time.

2 Audit Your Social Circle

Your habits are shaped by the people around you.

◈ **If your friends are active and eat healthy, you will too.**

⚠ **If your friends are lazy, eat junk, and complain, you will too.**

◈ **Find accountability partners.** Join a fitness group, online community, or challenge.

◈ **Follow people who inspire you.** Social media can help—if you follow the right people.

◈ **Cut out toxic influences.** If people pressure you to eat badly, drink excessively, or stay inactive, **distance yourself.**

You don't have to cut people out completely, but **you do have to protect your progress.**

3 Create Systems, Not Just Goals

Most people set goals like:

◈ **"I want to lose 20 pounds."**

◈ **"I want to eat better."**

◈ **"I want to exercise more."**

And then they fail because **they don't have a system in place.**

The Right Way to Do It:

◈ **"I will meal prep every Sunday to stay on track."**

◈ **"I will walk for 15 minutes after dinner every night."**

◈ **"I will do 10 push-ups before getting in the shower."**

◈ **Goals are the destination. Systems are the roadmap.** Without a system, **you'll never get there.**

The Rewards of Change: Energy, Clarity, Confidence, Longevity

At first, change is hard. But once you stick with it, **everything gets easier.**

Here's what happens when you commit:

� **More Energy**

� You wake up feeling **refreshed, not exhausted.**

� You don't need **caffeine to survive the day.**

� You actually feel like **moving instead of sitting all day.**

� **Mental Clarity**

�♂ Your mind is **sharper, faster, and more focused.**

� Brain fog disappears—you actually feel **present.**

� You retain information better, think clearly, and **make smarter decisions.**

� **Confidence & Strength**

� You feel **stronger**—physically and mentally.

� You stop feeling **self-conscious** about your body.

� You gain **self-discipline that carries over into every area of life.**

� **Longevity: More Years, Better Years**

� You **live longer, but more importantly—you live better.**

� You avoid hospitals, medications, and surgeries.

� You stay **independent and active**, instead of becoming a burden to your family.

Imagine a future where:

� You have the **energy to travel, play with your kids, and enjoy life.**

� You aren't **worried about hospital visits, medications, or disease.**

� You wake up **feeling good every single day.**

That's **the reward for staying consistent.**

No More Excuses: It's Time to Take Ownership

⚠ **It's not about being "too busy."**

⚠ **It's not about not having enough motivation.**

⚠ **It's not about waiting for the "right time."**

◈ **Excuses won't change your life.**

◈ **Action will.**

◈ **One step today. One choice today. One habit today.**

That's all it takes to change your future.

◈ **Start habit stacking.**

◈ **Clean up your environment.**

◈ **Surround yourself with the right influences.**

◈ **Stay consistent—even when you don't feel like it.**

Your future **is in your hands.**

Are you ready to fight for it?

◈ **Turn the page. Your transformation starts NOW.**

40

Chapter 7: What Happens If You Ignore This Book

◈ **This is your last warning.** ◈

By now, you know the truth. You know your health is in danger. You know that if you don't change, your body **will break down.**

You also know the **solution.** You've seen how simple changes—eating real food, moving your body, and shifting your mindset—can **save your life.**

But here's the problem: **Most people won't do it.**

Most people **will close this book and go right back to their old habits.** They'll tell themselves:

◈ "I'll start next week."

◈ "One more bad meal won't hurt."

◈ "I'm not that unhealthy."

And then, **life will catch up with them.**

They'll wake up one day, hooked up to machines in a hospital bed, **wishing they had listened.**

But by then, it'll be **too late.**

A Final Warning: The Pain, Regret, and Suffering Waiting Ahead

If you ignore this book, here's what your future looks like:

◈ **A sudden heart attack that could have been prevented.**

◈ **A stroke that leaves you unable to talk, move, or live independently.**

◈ **Diabetes that leads to blindness, kidney failure, or amputations.**

◈ **Years of suffering, medications, surgeries, and regret.**

This isn't a scare tactic. **It's reality.**

Millions of people **die every year from preventable diseases**—and every single one of them thought they had more time.

But they didn't.

The Harsh Truth: If You Don't Act NOW, You May Never Act at All

Here's something most people don't realize:

◈ **The longer you wait, the harder it gets.**

If you don't start eating healthier today, **you're even less likely to start next month.**

If you don't start moving today, **your body will get weaker, making it even harder later.**

If you don't take control today, **your excuses will pile up, trapping you in a cycle of failure.**

Before you know it...

◈ **You're on five medications.**

◈ **You're too sick to exercise.**

◈ **You're in and out of hospitals.**

◈ **You're running out of time.**

Every day you don't take action, **you're making a choice.**

You're choosing disease over health.

You're choosing regret over action.

You're choosing a slow, painful decline instead of taking control.

What's it going to take?

Will you wait until the pain is unbearable?

Will you wait until your body completely breaks down?

Will you wait until it's **too late to fix it?**

Or will you finally say **ENOUGH** and do something about it?

The Commitment Challenge: Will You Take Control of Your Life Today?

This is it. **Your moment of truth.**

You have **two choices right now:**

◈ **Choice 1:** Ignore this book. Keep eating the same foods, avoiding exercise, and making excuses. Keep hoping nothing bad happens—until it does.

OR

◈ **Choice 2:** Take control. Start today. Make one small change. Commit to your future health.

◈ **Not tomorrow. Not next week. Not when it's "convenient."**

◈ **TODAY.**

If You're Serious, Take This Challenge Right Now:

◈ **Write down ONE habit you'll start today.** (Example: "I will drink water instead of soda.")

◈ **Write down ONE reason why you refuse to stay the same.** (Example: "I want to live to see my grandkids grow up.")

◈ **Tell someone about your decision.** (Accountability makes all the difference.)

◈ **If you commit, your life will change.**

If you don't? You already know what's coming.

◈ **This is your last chance.**

Are you going to ignore this wake-up call, or are you going to fight for your life?

◈ **The choice is yours.**

Conclusion: Your Life is in Your Hands

◈ **No one is coming to save you.** ◈

Not your doctor.

Not your family.

Not some magic pill.

◈ **Only YOU can change your life.**

For years, you've been told that medication will fix it. That surgery will fix it. That there's always more time.

But that's a lie.

◈ **Time is running out.**

Every day you wait, you get weaker.

Every unhealthy meal takes a toll.

Every excuse pushes you closer to disease, disability, and death.

There's no "later." **There's only now.**

A Simple Choice: Change... or Suffer the Consequences

At this moment, **you stand at a crossroads.**

◈ **One path leads to regret.**

- Keep eating the same way.
- Keep avoiding exercise.
- Keep hoping your body doesn't give out.
- Keep watching your health decline.

One day, you'll wake up in a hospital bed, tubes in your arms, wondering why you didn't listen.

◈ **The other path leads to freedom.**

- You take action—today.
- You choose better food, one meal at a time.
- You move your body, even if it's just a few minutes a day.
- You refuse to be another statistic.

◈ **This isn't about "trying." It's about deciding.**

Deciding that you will fight for your life.

Deciding that you will no longer be a victim of your own habits.

Deciding that you are worth saving.

Your Future Begins Now

You've read the warnings.

You've seen what's at stake.

You know the consequences of doing nothing.

Now, **what will you do?**

⚠ Will you close this book and pretend you didn't read it?

⚠ Will you let excuses keep you trapped in an unhealthy life?

⚠ Will you wait until it's too late?

Or...

⟐ Will you take control?

⟐ Will you fight for your body, your energy, your future?

⟐ Will you prove to yourself—and to the world—that you will not go down without a fight?

⟐ **This is your moment. This is your life. This is your choice.**

⟐ **Change starts NOW.**

⟐ **Go. Take action. Fight for your future. You deserve it.**

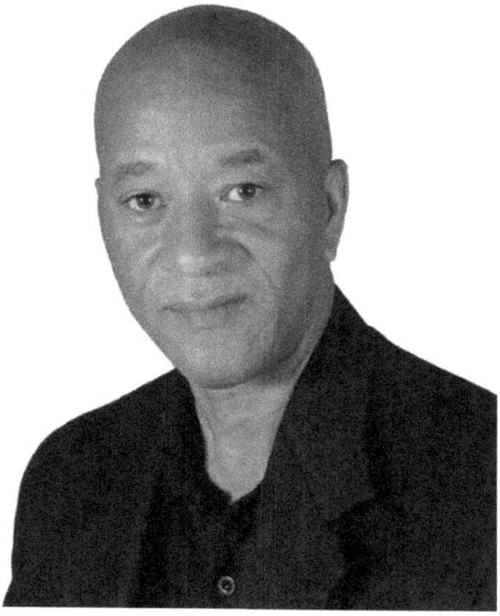

About the Author

Wayne C. Robinson is a U.S. Navy veteran, investigative journalist, and best-selling author who exposes hidden corruption in politics, media, and industry. His work challenges mainstream narratives and empowers readers with truth, transparency, and real solutions.

Read more at www.enemieswithinus.com.

www.ingramcontent.com/pod-product-compliance
Lightning Source LLC
LaVergne TN
LVHW050747061126
851857LV00013B/1038

"This is the last warning most people never hear."